GUIDE TO LUXURIOUS LONG HEALTHY HAIR

the natural way

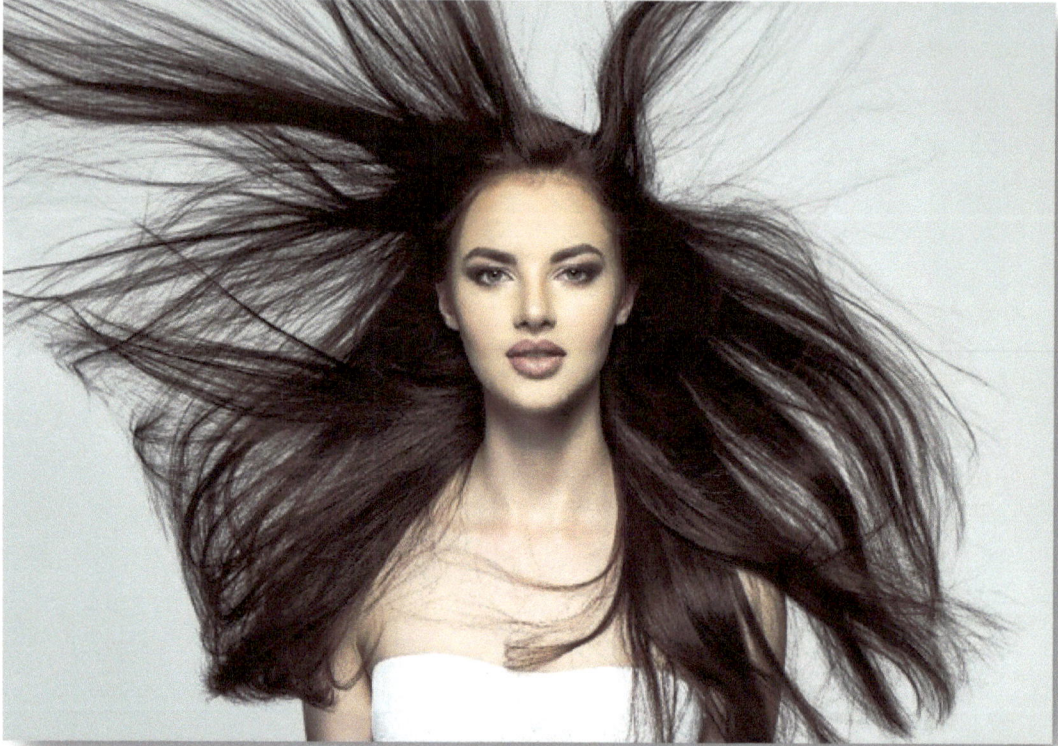

Indian Head Massage

Stephanie Marie Roberts

*Dedicated to all my past and present students. You have taught **me** much along the way.*

Stephanie

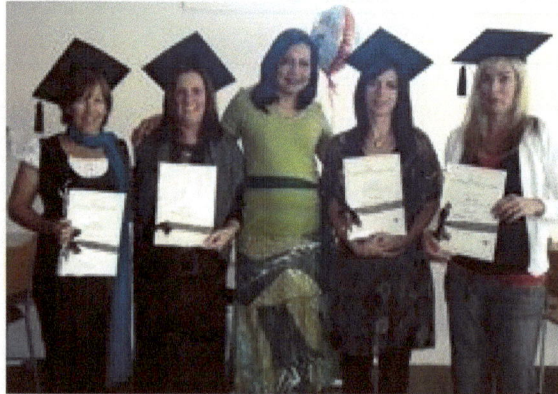

Live as if you were to die tomorrow. Learn as if you were to live forever.

~MAHATHMA GANDHI

FOREWORD

HAIR, Long, Luxurious and Healthy!

Ancient Natural Therapies: Time-Old Secrets

Discover the Healing Power of Traditional Techniques

Throughout the ages, humans have sought ways to heal and enhance their well-being using the natural resources available to them. Many ancient therapies have stood the test of time, offering remedies and enhancing beauty with their age-old secrets. Among these treasured techniques, Indian head massage stands out for its ability to promote beauty and ensure strong, healthy hair.

I'm an Indian born teacher of holistic and spiritual therapies and an internationally qualified beauty therapy teacher (ITEC, London) for over thirty years, having run two successful international colleges in Sydney and Canberra, Australia—*Stephanie Roberts' International Beauty Training College* and *Stephanie Roberts' Art of Beauty Training College*. Being of Indian heritage, I was the recipient of many Indian head massages as a child from my 'Dadi' (paternal grandmother). I have her to thank for my luxurious, long, raven-black hair today.

Indian Head Massage
Indian head massage, also known as Champissage, is a traditional practice that has been passed down through generations in India. This massage technique focuses on the head, neck, and shoulders, using a variety of movements to stimulate blood circulation, relieve tension, and promote relaxation.

Indian Head Massage promotes hair health. Regular Indian head massages can improve hair texture, reduce hair fall, and even stimulate hair growth. The increased blood circulation to the scalp ensures that hair follicles receive ample nutrients. By focusing on the upper body, Indian head massage helps to release accumulated tension and stress, leading to a sense of

1

overall well-being. The improved blood flow to the scalp and face can lead to a healthier complexion and a natural glow.

Indian head massage has both physical and psychological benefits. It helps soothe and relax the nervous system while relieving joint and muscle stiffness. And, of course, it is a very beneficial treatment for tension headaches and eyestrain. Different strokes and pressure are used to stimulate the lymphatic and circulatory system, which assist in removal of waste and toxins. These are just a few of the therapeutic benefits of this technique. It's a deep, relaxing therapy that rebalances the body's energy to produce a sense of peace, calm and well-being. It is believed that three of the main energy centres of the human body are found in the head: brow, crown and throat. Indian head massage stimulates these important energy centres (chakras) which help to maintain the body's balance of energy and a feeling of peace and tranquillity.

Follow through the instructions and repeat at least three to five times, till you become adept at the skill. It is a wonderful treatment for balancing mind and body. Your life will flow and bring you great peace and contentment if you practise this skill ... as well as BEAUTIFUL LUXURIOUS HEALTHY HAIR!

Table of Contents

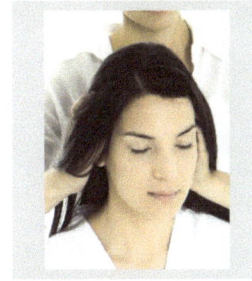

Introduction

What this course will teach you:

Indian head massage with treatment time from fifteen minutes to an hour.

* A massage where client remains fully clothed and in seated position.

* General massage and stretching techniques.

* Lymphatic drainage.

* Acupressure points.

* Energy balancing.

A massage with many therapeutic benefits:

* Relaxes nervous system.

* Relieves joint and muscle stiffness.

* Helps tension headaches and eyestrain.

* Stimulates circulatory and lymphatic system.

* Helps general stress and tension.

* A beauty treatment for the face and hair.

* Oil blend for relaxation, stimulation and improvement of condition of hair.

Who this course is for:

* Lay person wanting to treat friends and relatives.

* Professional massage therapist wanting to learn further techniques.

* Beauty therapist and hairdresser wanting to learn new techniques.

* Anybody wanting a relaxing and healing time to be nurtured and cleansed.

ON AIR at Radio Station 93.3 FM

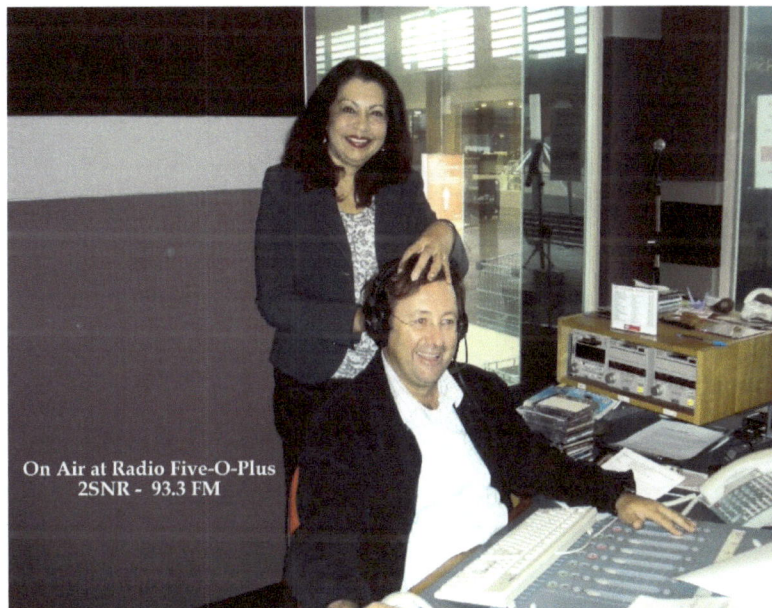

On Air at Radio Five-O-Plus
2SNR - 93.3 FM

History of Indian Head Massage

An Indian head massage will energise your mind and allow tension to slip away. This ancient technique has been practised for over a thousand years in India, being passed down from generation to generation. It is both therapeutic and a beauty treatment with many wonderful benefits. Indian head massage can be given almost anywhere. The receiver remains fully clothed seated in a chair or can sit cross legged on the ground. It involves using a sequence of moves such as energy-balancing techniques, lymphatic drainage, stimulating acupressure points, stretching and general massage to the shoulders, neck, face and scalp. The techniques work on both the physical and ethereal level.

If you are confused about what all this might involve first you should know that all of this is completely painless. We only discuss lymphatic drainage and acupressure points to indicate *where* and *what* will be happening for you during the process.

Acupressure points: Imagine putting cookie dough in a freezer. When you take it out it is hard, but you begin kneading and massaging it with your hands and eventually it loosens and softens back to its original state. That is the basis of what the masseuse will do for you during the procedure. Stress, anxiety, sleep deprivation, and even sitting down in an office chair all day can cause the muscles in your head to harden and tighten. It is important to know where on your head those muscles overlap so they can be massaged out to allow more blood flow and tension relief.

Lymphatic Drainage: It may not be the most attractive sounding procedure, but it happens without us doing a thing. All you, as the client, have to do is sit and let the masseuse do their healing. The draining is basically in the lymph nodes around your throat and the entire lymphatic system. Massaging out any blockage or fluid-based interference helps in a variety

6

of ways. This includes, but is not limited to: detoxification, tissue regeneration, and strengthening the immune system. This is important because, while lymph nodes can *survive* while under duress, they do not *thrive*. Leaving them unattended for an extended time can cause severe health issues all over the body. Lymph node drainage is incredibly important for surviving and recovering cancer patients.

Think of it as a full mind massage. Not only are your senses kicking in on the outside, but you are feeling the changes on the inside too. Therapists or masseuses who plan to give you the experience of a lifetime are going to be bringing about the balance of your mind and body. This will include your mind, your chakras, and your hair follicles. You will feel the change in your entire body. It will invigorate and revive three main chakras, the throat chakra, the head chakra, and the crown chakra. They all encompass one thing: your mind. This clears up critical thinking. For many years we did not have the medicine to heal sicknesses or anxiety. People went to healers when they needed help. These healers did exactly what you will read here. This age-old method is resurfacing in the world as more people turn away from the over-medicated and over-diagnosed practices.

Indian head massage is a beauty treatment as well. The secret of Indian women's lustrous, shining hair is the mixture of oils and the special blend of aromatherapy oils used to relax or energise the person. (Oil on hair is optional, of course.) It also is like a mini facial, minimising fine lines and replenishing skin from within.

A short treatment of fifteen minutes can be given or, for more profound results, treatments can take up to an hour. It is a great technique that is easy to learn for the professional therapist or lay person wanting to treat friends and relatives.

Indian head massage was originally developed by women who practised the techniques within their family. My grandmother set up this ritual every morning for me when I stayed with her as a child in her wonderful, terraced home in Poona, India. Out on the terrace we would sit, under the jamun tree. I loved this fruit, shaped like a grape, with a soft, dark-purple, almost black skin and a lighter purple flesh. When eaten, the fruit coats the mouth and the tongue with deep purple for a few hours.

My lips and tongue would be stained with the purple berry juice, which ran deliciously down my chin as Nana Lily oiled and massaged my long black hair. A head bath, as she called it, would follow, with ladles of hot water scooped out of a wooden bucket and hard scrubbing. I almost felt she'd scrub my head off sometimes, but the stimulation of follicles must have given me the beautiful, thick, strong dark hair I still own today. The use of oil today is optional, but I do recommend it, as it can play an important role in improving the lustre and condition of the hair.

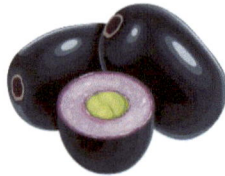

If you are only looking for irresistible hair, you should still read this book through to see what other amazing benefits you will receive. Let us begin discussing the procedure. It is easy to do at home. There is no need to go to a salon or clinic and pay half your paycheque to get the benefits. I want you to feel as free and liberated as I am with my hair routine. You have a right to the best hair possible for you.

Physical and Psychological Benefits

Indian head massage has both physical and psychological benefits. It helps soothe and relax the nervous system while relieving joint and muscle stiffness. And, of course, it is a very beneficial for tension headaches and eyestrain. Different strokes and pressure are used to stimulate the lymphatic and circulatory system, which assist in removal of waste and toxins. These are just a few of the therapeutic benefits of this technique. It's a deep, relaxing therapy that rebalances the body's energy to produce a deep sense of peace, calm and well-being. Three of the main energy centres (chakras) of the human body are found in the head: brow, crown and throat. Indian head massage stimulates these important energy centres, which help to maintain the body's balance of energy and a feeling of peace and tranquillity.

All the chakras are explained in detail in my *Crystal Healing Workshop*. I will also be publishing a workshop on chakra healing.

If you are not already familiar with chakras, imagine a flower. There are the petals of the flower and the stem that holds it up. That is what these chakras are for your mind and body. The crown chakra that rests on the top of your head is the main flower. Around it are the throat and 'third-eye' chakras, that finish the flower, and the stem leads down your spine and out through your feet. Seven chakras work together to keep your life liveable. In this book we are going to focus on the main parts of your flower, perhaps the most important. We will give you insight into how to change your wilting body into a flourishing blossom.

The intuitive chakra or brow chakra is sometimes called the 'third eye' or 'sixth sense'. It is located on the forehead, between and slightly above the eyebrows.

If strong, you have the ability to make accurate decisions about your life and your career, and see other people as they are. You know things and have a clear sense of direction and clarity in everything you do. You can visualise where your life is headed. Others rely on you for guidance and advice.

If weak, you are indecisive and feel helpless, always looking to others for their opinions about yourself. You feel spiritually lost and suffer with tension headaches or migraines.

It is important that this be revitalised because it thinks of the rights and wrongs of decisions. It can think critically through a variety of outcomes and help you determine which life-changing choices to make. It is nicknamed the 'third-eye' because it focuses on intuition and awareness. That is not something you want slacking during work, life, or relationships.

The crown chakra is located in the crown of the head.

If strong, you feel connected to a higher power, whether God, the Universe or your Higher Self. You feel protected and watched over. You feel gratitude for your life, appreciation for what you have, and love and compassion for others. People describe you as a happy and glowing individual.

If weak, you feel very much alone in this world and unworthy of spiritual guidance. You may feel angry that your higher power has abandoned you, and you often suffer from migraines and tension headaches.

The crown keeps you motivated. You know there is a goal to reach, and you appreciate every step of the way. Your confidence soars because you are not worried about the social anxieties of the day. This chakra is responsible for your drive. It is what makes you do what you want to do, and enables you to visualise it in order to *do* it. You will feel when this chakra is blocked.

Everything will seem so far away. You will feel as though nothing you do is ever right or correct. After you take care of this chakra you'll quickly feel the change in mentality.

The throat chakra is located at the base of the throat where the collarbone comes into a 'V'. It is the centre of speech and communication. It's important to remember, however, that communication is not just about talking—it's also about listening.

If strong, you have a strong voice and can voice your opinions, thoughts and emotions. You speak the truth, even if it is uncomfortable to some. You are admired for your willpower and strong communication skills. You can express yourself well—and this expression isn't always verbal.

If weak, you feel you have nothing of importance to say and frequently settle to follow other people's opinions. You often suffer with a blocked and sore throat. Other signs of imbalance are lying, arrogance, talking too much, being manipulative, fear and timidity. When you feel a 'lump in your throat' during sadness, this is a physical expression of how some of your emotions are stored in the base of your throat. The ears and shoulders are also associated with this chakra, so physical discomforts can arise when this chakra is out of balance.

As humans our lives are blessed with hundreds of different ways to communicate. But what if the way and reason you communicate is restricted or gone? You'll notice this chakra is weak only when you've had a chance to re-energise it. This chakra can hide its problems in secret forms. Communication is vital for all forms of life and success. Even those who have no voice strive to communicate. You should strive to communicate in the best possible way. It is your right, and you deserve to have your voice heard.

Nervous System Benefits

Indian head massage relieves joint and muscle stiffness, even if it is from an old injury or recurring back pain. It can be used as a physical therapy of sorts. It helps relieve tension headaches and eyestrain. Ocular muscles connect throughout your head. When your eyes are constantly focusing on a screen, or squinting at a book or board in front of you, it causes your muscles to tense and harden. Think of it as a rubber band. You strain your eyes to see and focus, but when the rubber band is pulled too far, it can sometimes fail to return to its normal state. When you work on a computer for long periods of time, you should take a break every twenty minutes or so and stare across the room at the furthest thing you see. This maintains the muscle strength and strong focus. Indian head massage stimulates both the circulatory and lymphatic system. It also helps relieve general stress and tension. Lastly it is a beauty treatment for the face and hair. The list goes on, but this should already be enough to convince you of the value of a trial.

As with all healing methods, some patients might need to verify their health beforehand. Please check the list below carefully. If you are unsure about whether or not you qualify for this, ask a qualified masseuse or physician/healer.

Indian head massage is very safe, but there are a few instances when it should not be performed. When you

* suffer from low or high blood pressure;

* have a high temperature or any feeling of unwellness;

* have gastric problems, especially food poisoning;

* have injuries or surgery involving the head, neck or upper back;

* have localised skin disorders or bruising in the area;

* are under the influence of alcohol;

* have infectious diseases or inflammatory conditions in the area.

Other notes and precautions:

Those with arthritis or bone degenerative diseases (osteoporosis) may require a softer/calmer massage.

The amount of pressure will depend on the age or tolerance of the person receiving the massage.

Be sure to allow your body time to readjust after the massage before going. This will allow the toxins that have been released to fully exit the body.

Closing

There are many reasons to try Indian head massage. Even if you only want a massage to strengthen and regenerate your hair follicles, you will still receive the added mental benefits. This is an easy and painless procedure that you can do fully clothed.

The chakras work together throughout your body. The three within the head region deal with memory, emotions, thoughts, and motivation. Each has a specific job, but they work simultaneously together. In the procedure section of this book we will find each chakra's position, so you know when and where it can be activated. You will be able to feel the flood of vitalities almost immediately. However, as with any procedure, there might be side effects. I have listed these throughout the book so you know exactly what to expect. It is important for the client and therapist to be completely transparent. I put everything on the table here. You can also contact me directly should you have any additional questions. I love being a constant recipient of both the Indian scalp treatment and the Indian head massage, so much so that I learned the procedure and perfected it to share with you.

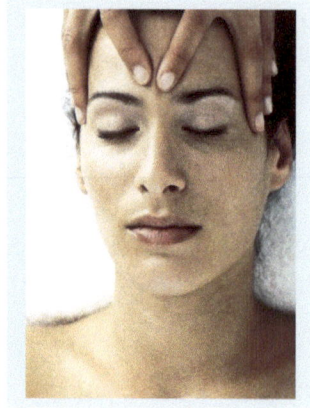

Indian Herbal Scalp Treatment

This treatment promotes circulation, healthy scalp, hair growth and prevents loss of hair. Please remember that nothing happens in a day. This treatment works best when it has become a habit. It takes around twenty-one days to develop a true habit, but you will see results in as little as two weeks. Remember to keep consistent.

The health of hair, skin, and nails show the true health of a person. Before it was known that genetics contributes to premature baldness or fragile hair, it was believed the damage resulted from an unhealthy diet or routine. They relied on oils and herbs from nature to help keep their hair looking healthy and strong. This is still widely practised today, and hair has never looked stronger. I have written out a recipe and 'ingredient' list so you can go right to the store. If you are unable to find any of these ingredients, message me personally with any questions. I provide the recipe below, and you can go to your local health food store or essential oil provider.

Materials Required:

Plastic bowl.

Hairdressing tint brush.

Indian herbal oil. (You can purchase this in a good Asian grocery shop.) If you can't find it, write to me personally. Or use my personal 'Hair Regrowth Remedy' oil mixture, as given in my recipe below.

Atomiser.

Rosewater 100 ml. Blend with five drops rosemary and five drops lavender, and fill atomiser with blend.

Method and Procedure:

Protect clothing with towel.

Part hair in sections and spray with blend in atomiser.

Part hair in sections and apply warm herbal oil to scalp, section by section.

Cover hair with disposable cap or wrap in glad wrap.

Sit under steamer for ten to fifteen minutes or wrap head with hot towel compress, changing the towel three times as it cools.

Perform Indian head massage.

Label your bottles of spray. Here is an example of one to stick on your bottle of spray:

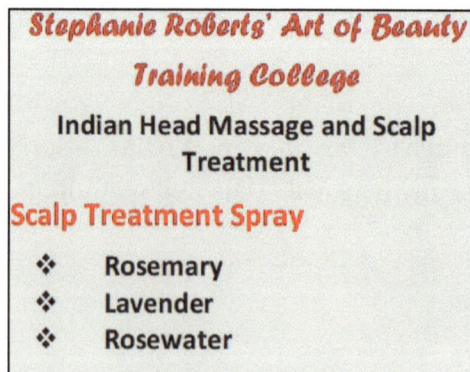

Stephanie Roberts' Art of Beauty

Training College

Indian Head Massage and Scalp Treatment

Scalp Treatment Spray

- ❖ **Rosemary**
- ❖ **Lavender**
- ❖ **Rosewater**

Leave oil in hair for two to three hours or overnight if possible for maximum benefit.

Or:

Wash hair with herbal shampoo and conditioner.

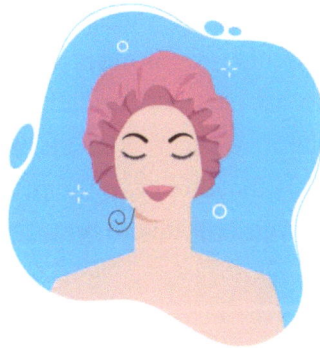

Oil and Head

There are many products on the market today that claim they can grow hair. For those who suffer with hair loss problems, these expensive products can be tempting. However, some are natural, less expensive and have a better success rate. It is not a quick fix. It may take up to six months to see good results, so be persistent and you will be rewarded with healthy strong hair.

Essential Oils

I could write an entire book about using oils in your life, but we are going to focus on those that benefit your mind and hair. Before we had shampoos and conditioners, what did people do to 'freshen up' their hair? They used oils from flowers, seeds, plants, lemon peels, and more. These oils became the foundation of most perfumes and cleaning products worldwide. Almost every cleaning product or hair supplement contains some sort of essential oil. However, the oils are most likely diluted in chemicals that can have the reverse affect. So, when it comes to finding a trustworthy way to increase your hair health, you should go right to the source of the essential oils.

Rosemary Oil

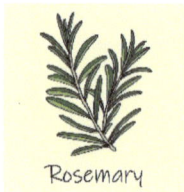

Rosemary stimulates the hair follicles. This in turn encourages hair growth—not only longer, but stronger. It also helps with flaky or dry scalps, colouration of grey hairs, and premature balding or hair loss.

Jojoba Oil

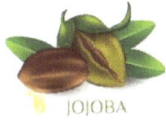

Jojoba oil is very good to loosen dead scales and remove crusted build up on the scalp. This build up blocks the hair follicles, slowing down hair growth.

Lavender Oil

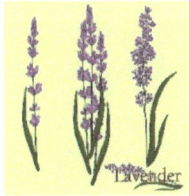

Lavender oil is my favourite. I use it for insect bites, itches of all kinds, rejuvenation of the skin, headaches or for a good night's sleep. Studies have also shown that people suffering from alopecia (hair loss), who massaged their heads daily with lavender and other essential oils, developed quite significant hair growth over a period of six months.

Coconut Oil

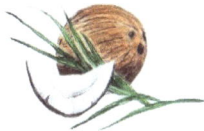

Coconut oil is one of India's favourite oils. It nourishes hair and gives it a beautiful shine. It keeps lice and dandruff at bay and encourages re-growth and repair of damaged hair.

Thyme Oil

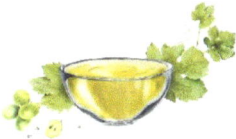

Thyme oil improves circulation to the scalp. Massage it in well. Thyme provides hair with beautiful shine, lustre, fullness and bounce.

Hair Regrowth Remedy

Mix:

three drops of lavender

two drops of thyme

two drops of rosemary

4 tsp. grape seed oil (this is the base oil or carrier oil)

1/2 tsp. jojoba oil

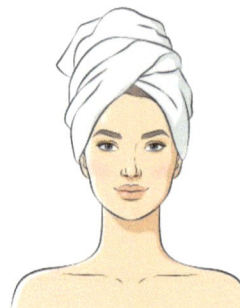

Perform Indian head massage or just massage into scalp for two minutes.

Wrap a warm towel around your head to increase absorption or use a steamer.

Wash your hair with an Indian herbal shampoo after one hour or leave overnight. Put a towel on your pillow to absorb excess. If you are sleeping alone that night, you can try this!

Do this daily for up to six months. Remember: perseverance! You will be rewarded.

Label your bottle of oil. Here is an example of a label to stick on your bottle:

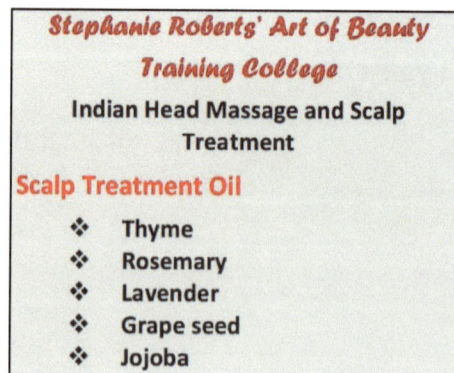

Stephanie Roberts' Art of Beauty Training College

Indian Head Massage and Scalp Treatment

Scalp Treatment Oil

- ❖ Thyme
- ❖ Rosemary
- ❖ Lavender
- ❖ Grape seed
- ❖ Jojoba

Indian Head Massage

Introduction

Good health depends on balanced energy. This energy, called 'chi' or 'ki' in Oriental medicine or 'prana' in Indian tradition is the Life Force itself. It permeates our bodies and every living thing in the universe. When our energy is unbalanced we feel out of sorts or unwell. Balancing energy has been practised for over a thousand years in India, and now it is practised worldwide.

Stress, poor diet, strong emotions or toxin build-up are all symptoms of modern living that can unbalance life energy and create areas of negativity. The power of energy healing lies in rebalancing the Life Force so that the flow of energy within us is constant, effortless and unblocked. Traditional Indian head massage affects the pulsing rhythms of cerebrospinal fluid, carrying healing messages around the body and stimulating the body's self-healing mechanisms.

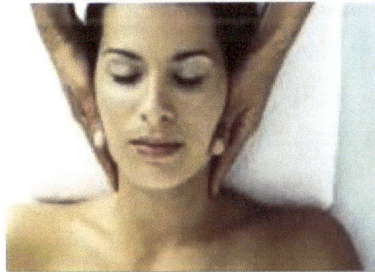

21

Tension in the muscles is released, dispersing toxins, reducing mental and physical stress and improving blood flow to the brain.

Life energy flows within us and, by working on the channels it flows through, or specific points or areas, this energy can be brought into balance.

There are several reasons why a person might want to seek out an Indian head massage:

*   Migraines (both head and optic)

*   Stress (emotional/mental)

*   Sinus pressure

*   Office related pain (air-conditioning/fluorescent lights)

*   Cell-phone radiation

*   Posture (from slouching in front of a computer or driving)

Unfortunately, you might relate to one or more of the above. That could be why you are reading my book today. You want to know how to rid yourself of the pain for good. If you are not already convinced, let me give you another recap of what this massage will offer you, and then we will start digging deep into the preparation and procedure.

The Indian head massage will help with:

*   increasing glucose and oxygen to the brain;

*   increasing circulation;

*   dispersing toxins and blockage;

* stimulating hair follicles and promoting hair growth;

* improving concentration;

* relieving sinus pressure.

Let us now begin understanding exactly what is involved.

Preparation (What to Expect)

The main goal of the therapist will be to restore balance and harmony within your mind and body. They are going to be relieving the tension in the three higher chakras in your body, so their goal is to ensure you are comfortable enough to give them access. During the massage, you may notice that you feel pressure or touch on other parts of your body besides the head. That is called reflexology massage. The therapist uses the many acupressure points around your neck and head to access other parts of your body.

Indian head massage has a few main focuses. It seeks to balance emotional, physical, and mental stress. The therapist will increase the blood flow to the head and brain. You should be able to feel the effects of this almost immediately after the massage.

Traditional Indian head massage is delivered with the client seated. However, some people prefer to be massaged lying down. With the client in a seated position it is very easy to reach all areas of the head, neck and shoulders. A professional massage chair is best; however, a good straight-backed chair will suffice.

The client remains clothed. Just remove extra clothing such as a jumper or jacket.

Drape towel around the shoulders of the client.

If a professional massage chair is used, prepare the breathing hole by wiping with antiseptic and laying disposable paper or a clean hand towel around the aperture. The client will rest the head (face down) into the opening.

If a standard chair is used, position the client comfortably, sitting erect, spine well supported by the back of the chair.

If Indian scalp treatment is incorporated into Indian head massage, the client will have had warm herbal oil infused into the scalp prior to the massage. You will work with the oil in the scalp. No oil should be applied to the back, neck and shoulders. Remember that the client is fully clothed, and any oil applied to the back, neck and shoulders would soil her clothing.

This technique should be used in a slow, meditative way. Use one or more fingers, your thumbs, and the heel of the hand or your whole hand. These movements stimulate circulation, move stagnant blood and energy, and tone and loosen the muscles. The rotations also stimulate the scalp and improve hair growth.

What to expect (after first massage)

Soreness: Depending on the location or tightness of your muscles, there could be a small amount of ache or pain the day after the massage. This is due to the blood flow and increased circulation. When you receive a massage, or apply pressure where things are normally tense, it causes blood flow. If you have been able to walk around with a tight and out of place back for a long time, it is because your body has adapted to it, and not in a good way. When we are constantly slouching or carrying weight the wrong way, our muscles become attuned to it. Eventually, after enough time has passed, you won't be able to feel that pain because the blood has stopped circulating to it. People can go years with back pain their mind has just 'adapted' too. That is why there will be a few aches and pains after the neck or shoulder massage. The head massage can relax muscles you did not realise were tight.

Drink water: Now that blood is recirculating through your body, you'll want to stay hydrated to give yourself the most benefit. Keep your blood vessels wide and hydrated so the blood flow can continue without restraint.

Avoid caffeine or alcohol: As your blood is now flowing freely through your head, you might find you are less tolerant to caffeine or alcohol, so try to avoid them as best you can for at least a little while.

Flu-like symptoms: This is a potential side effect from the lymph-node drainage and/or the sinus-pressure drainage. This may be nausea, or a slight headache due to the toxins now flowing freely through your body. It should only last half a day or so, and usually the first massage is the worst as the blockage is usually rather severe.

Exhaustion: Even though you were just sitting in a chair the entire time, you might feel the urge to nap or rest. This is also part of the toxin drainage, but also has to do with the blood flow and activity that is now awake inside your body. Your chakras have been reactivated. They are replenished from a long, coma-like state. This would be exhausting for anyone. You also took your head on a roller-coaster ride, and it might just want to relax for a little while. Feel free to take a five- or ten-minute cat-nap, but too much longer may result in trouble sleeping—an elevation of the exhaustion.

Emotional: As I stated before: toxin release. This also includes stress release. You know that feeling when you are holding back tears or anger? How sometimes when you finally let yourself cry it is a wild explosion of tears and chaos? That is exactly what the therapist will do for you. They will massage out the emotional tension, and it can make you feel a little emotionally unstable for a moment or two. This is completely normal, and the therapist will encourage you to let those emotions pass through, instead of trying to block or hold them back again.

You will find almost instant relief after your second session. I cannot express enough how important it is to STAY CONSISTENT in your head-massage routine. Not only for beautiful, strong hair, but for your health as well.

Indian Head Massage Procedure

NOTE: This pattern is to be adhered to in all the following sequences where it says, 'general pattern'. Keep referring to this. I suggest you write it down so you can easily refer to it whilst learning. Soon you won't need it. You'll be an expert! Many have been helped and healed by Indian head massage. It is a wonderful, balancing treatment. This will all become muscle memory after a few practices, but always refer to the notes if you get lost or confused. A head massage can have incredible benefits, as long as it is delivered precisely.

The General Pattern:

* Support the client's forehead with your right hand.

* Work in lines.

* Work with your left hand.

* Commence on hairline—work left half of head, ending at nape of neck.

* Work approximately two finger widths apart in parallel lines.

* Change hands.

* Support the client's forehead with your left hand.

* Repeat the same pattern on the right half of head.

Head

This technique should be used in a slow, meditative way. Use one or more fingers, your thumbs, and the heel of the hand or your whole hand.

These movements stimulate circulation, move stagnant blood and energy, and tone and loosen the muscles. The rotations also stimulate the scalp and improve hair growth. Remember to follow the general pattern.

One finger rotations:

*   Use middle or index finger.

*   Place pad or finger into centre of forehead and hairline.

*   Use firm pressure, rotate fingers for three to five seconds.

*   Follow general pattern (i.e. two fingers' width apart).

*   Complete left half of head.

*   Complete right half of head.

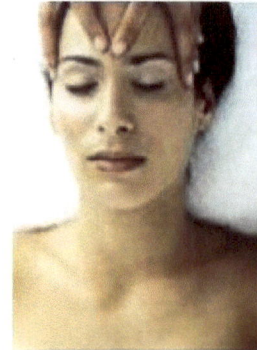

Two finger or four finger rotations:

*   Support forehead with your right hand.

* Work rotations centre of head with your left hand—hairline to the nape of the neck. Follow general pattern.

* Work sides of head with both your hands—hairline to just above ears. Follow general pattern.

Heel of hand rotations:

* Support forehead with your right hand.

* Place heel of your left hand at the nape of the neck and rotate, using small, gentle movements.

* Work up middle of head and over the top to the forehead. Follow general pattern.

* Work left side of head—nape of neck to front of head. Follow general pattern.

* Support forehead with your left hand.

* Work right side of head—nape of neck to front of head. Follow general pattern.

Pressure:

For this technique you can use one or more fingers. Particularly effective in treating stress and tension headaches. It also balances and boosts energy levels and subtly corrects pressure imbalances in the cerebrospinal fluid.

* Support head with your right hand.

* Start in the middle of hairline.

* Work with your left hand.

29

* Use one or more fingers to apply a firm pressure for three to five seconds then release.

* Work left side of head. Follow general pattern.

* Support head with your left hand.

* Work right side of head. Follow general pattern.

Rolling:

Rolling relaxes the mind and body, tones the scalp and eases tension. Use the outside edge of your hands rolling along the line of the little fingers with a constant flowing rhythm.

* Work with both your hands simultaneously.

* Commence at the centre of head.

* With your fingers straight, use the outside edge of the heels of your hands to make contact with the sides of the head. Now roll the pressure up the edges of your hands to the tips of your fingers. Roll back down to the heels of the hands.

* Maintain a smooth rhythm. Follow general pattern.

* For a stronger treatment, roll with one hand at a time, supporting the head with the other.

Knuckling:

This technique uses the knuckles. This is a vigorous and stimulating treatment which boosts energy levels and encourages deeper breathing.

* Work with both hands simultaneously.

* Make hands into fists.

* Rotate fingers, knuckles rolling into scalp.

* Commence at the middle of the head and work outwards to nape of the neck. Follow general pattern.

* Support forehead with left hand.

* Work centre panel of head. Work with the right hand, knuckling from forehead to nape of neck. Follow general pattern.

Tapping:

This is a technique that uses all the fingers. Tapping is vigorous and stimulating.

* Work with both hands simultaneously.

* Hold your hands so your fingertips are level.

* Keep your wrists loose.

* Press pads of fingers into scalp and bounce off rapidly with quick, light, smooth movements.

* Keep a regular rhythm. Follow general pattern.

Hair Pulling; Clapping; Vibrations:

Work with both hands simultaneously.

1. **Pulling**

*   Work with both hands simultaneously.

*   Comb your fingers lightly through hair to loosen it.

*   Commence on either side of neck and work to forehead.

*   Slide fingers up into hair, fingers apart, keeping close to scalp.

*   Gather a handful of hair. Close your fingers firmly and pull away from the head, allowing the hair to draw through your fingers under tension, creating a strong, even pull.

*   Repeat all over the head, always pulling the hair at right angles away from the scalp. Follow general pattern.

*   An alternate way of 'pulling' is to wrap a small section of hair around your finger and hold firmly for three to five seconds and release.

2. **Clapping**

*   Eases tense muscles, loosens stiffness in head.

*   Work with both hands cupped together.

*   Loose fingers and wrists.

*   Move in light percussion movements over whole head three to five seconds.

3. **Vibrations**

*   Relaxes the mind and body.

* Hold forehead with left hand.

* Work with right hand.

* Press palm against head near occipital hollow (hollow near centre of base of skull).

* Stiffen your hand to elbow and vibrate. Repeat movement three times.

* Finger rotation into occipital hollow to finish.

Neck, Ears, Eyes

NECK
Keeps the neck supple and eases tension.

* Support side of head with your left hand.

* Clench fist of your right hand and beat with your knuckles on the opposite side, neck down to shoulders three times.

* Support side of head with your right hand.

* Clench fist of your left hand and beat with your knuckles on the opposite side of neck down to shoulders three times.

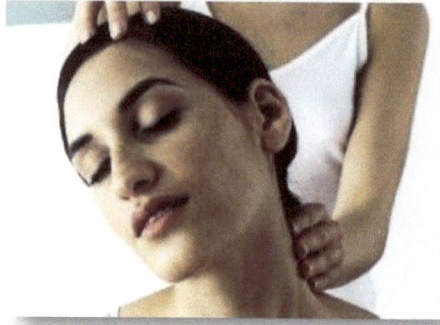

EARS

There are many acupuncture points in the ears. Using pressure and massage on these points balances the energy in the body and internal organs and in the mind and spirit. After this technique, the client may find her hearing is clearer and she feels brighter and more energetic.

Step 1:

* Start at the top of the ears where the ears join the head.

* Work with both your hands simultaneously.

* Work both ears simultaneously.

* Pinch the outside ridge hard, pulling the ears away from the head, and massage slowly with rotations for three to five seconds. Release and move one finger width and repeat.

* Continue all around ears to finish at the lobe.

Step 2:

* Grasp ear lobes firmly between index finger and thumb, pull down towards shoulders. Hold for three to five seconds and release.

* Grasp top of ears firmly between index finger and thumb, pull upwards. Hold for three to five seconds and release.

Step 3:

* Use index finger inside and your thumb behind ear to pinch and massage all the ridges, nooks and crannies firmly.

* Repeat Step 1 to finish.

EYES

The eyes contain many muscles, and giving them a good workout can improve sight. Short sight, long sight, astigmatism, and some focusing problems can all be helped by exercise and massage.

Step 1:

* Move to front of client.

* Work with both your hands.

* Hold one hand at full arm's length and the other about half way.

* Ask client to focus on one hand and then the other, moving quickly between them for a count of twenty.

Step 2:

* Finger rotations gently on the bridge of nose, using one finger rotations. Hold two to three seconds and release.

* Ask client to focus on finger, crossing eyes.

* Work down to tip of nose.

* Repeat twice.

* Ask client to close eyes and place his/her palms over them.

Step 3:

* With client's palms over eyes ask client to tense and release muscles to count of twenty.

* Tell client to feel heat and energy from palms relaxing the eyes.

Shoulders/Back

These carry a lot of tensions and burdens.

BACK

Thumb Rotations:

* Work with both hands simultaneously.

* Use pads of thumbs either side of spine, level with the base of the shoulder blades, and rotate firmly three to five seconds and release. Work to the edge of back horizontally. Follow general pattern.

* Work up to base of neck.

* Work up neck, to base of skull. Follow general pattern.

Heel of hand rotations:

* Work with both hands simultaneously.

* Use heel of hands either side of spine, level with the base of the shoulder blades, and rotate using strong pressure and small movements, three to five seconds. Work to edge of back horizontally. Follow general pattern.

* Work up to shoulders.

* For stronger pressure, brace client with your arm across front of shoulders and use one hand to work half of back. Change hands and repeat on the other half of back.

Hacking:

Hacking on the back and shoulders loosens the muscles and encourages deep breathing.

Work with both hands simultaneously.

Relax wrists. Beat with side of each hand alternatively in a light chopping action and keeping a regular rhythm.

SHOULDERS

Step 1:

* Work with both hands simultaneously.

* Place elbows on tops of shoulders, close to base of neck.

* Raise hands back towards you, leaning your body weight onto the shoulders. Hold for three to five seconds.

* Release the pressure, dropping your hands forward again.

* Move out to tops of arms. Repeat. Follow general pattern.

Step 2:

* Work with both hands simultaneously.

* With your hands held in loose fists, rest the back of your forearms on the tops of the shoulders, close to the base of the neck. Lean down firmly and hold for three to five seconds. Rock back your body to release. Move to top of shoulders. Follow general pattern.

Step 3:

* Hacking as for back.

* Total time for massage: thirty minutes

To Finish:

* Compress shoulders and back.

* Pressure point face and forehead.

* Stroke through hair.

Closing Thoughts

So now you have more knowledge than yesterday, and I hope you continue learning about this powerful health benefit and life-changing experience. You will see that even your memory is improved, and all those forgotten items on your shopping list will finally be remembered. My Indian heritage has blessed me with this knowledge, and it is something that is both a career and passion. I have encountered several sceptics, but have been happy to show them exactly what this medicine can provide. If you are ever feeling confused or have any questions at all my contact information is within the book.

Reminders:

Please remember to drink plenty of water before and after treatment, as your body is going to be circulating quite well, and those tight places will be taking in more than before.

It is completely normal to be sore or achy the day after, as the therapist has just awoken parts of your body that had become numb over the course of time.

You will feel re-energised in a matter of days, and I would love to hear your experience and success stories if you are willing to share. Life is important, and we only have one chance to really fulfil it. I have chosen to fulfil mine by sharing my experiences and practices with you and other readers all over the world. If my books give you happiness or peace, it will mean my passion has finally made a full circle. Thank you again for being part of this experience, and good luck with all of your endeavours throughout life and love.

Blessed be

♥

About the Author

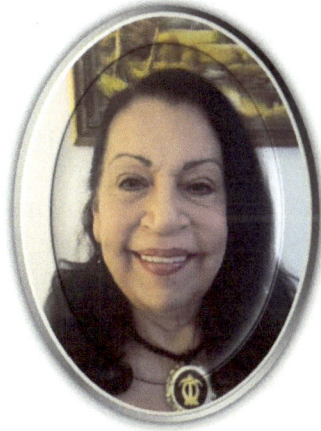

Stephanie Marie Roberts' love of writing has found a vibrant expression in illustrated children's books. Her journey as an author began with a simple yet profound desire to bring joy to her little grandsons, Joshua, Liam, and Nicky. What started as personal tales for her grandchildren blossomed into a passion for creating enchanting stories for children around the globe.

Stephanie's talent and dedication to her craft have been recognized through prestigious accolades. She is a proud recipient of the Book Excellence Literary Award and a Silver Medallist for her beloved books, "Liam Shark Boy" and "Joshua's World". These stories captivate young readers with their whimsical illustrations and heartwarming narratives.

Her literary repertoire extends beyond these award-winning titles. "Nicky Superhero" is a delightful tale embodying lessons in kindness and encouragement, inspiring children to embrace their inner hero. Meanwhile, "Billie Red Wattle Bird" is a charming story that imparts valuable lessons about responsibility and highlights the beauty of the Australian flora and fauna.

Stephanie's creative talents are not confined to children's literature alone. An incurable romantic at heart, she has also penned the touching fiction novel, "Always". This tear-jerking story draws from her own life experiences in the fifties and seventies, offering readers a poignant glimpse into a bygone era.

As Stephanie embarks on the final chapter of her life's narrative, she continues to define herself as a multifaceted writer. Her interests have expanded to encompass holistic studies. Her eLearning courses on Udemy are complemented by her insightful books, "Gain Insight to Read Tarot for Yourself in 5 Days" and "Healthy Relationships – The Well of True Gestures". These works serve as invaluable companions for those seeking to deepen their understanding of the Tarot and foster Healthy Relationships.

For those eager to delve into Stephanie's enchanting world of storytelling and holistic wisdom, her works can be found on her website and on Udemy. Stephanie Marie Roberts' journey as an author is a testament to her boundless creativity, her love for sharing stories, and her commitment to guiding others on their paths to self-discovery.

www.ingramcontent.com/pod-product-compliance
Lightning Source LLC
Chambersburg PA
CBHW060831270326
41933CB00002B/52